# ACETAMINOPHEN: HOW-TO-GUIDE

Understanding One of the World's Most Common Pain Relievers

**Dr. Mario Kjaer**

# Table of Contents

## CHAPTER ONE ............................................................................ 3
### Introduction .............................................................................. 3
### Early Origins ............................................................................. 4
### The Birth of Acetaminophen ................................................... 8
### Mechanism of Action ............................................................. 13
### Therapeutic Uses of Acetaminophen .................................... 22
### Co-administration with Other Medications ......................... 26

## CHAPTER TWO ........................................................................ 29
### Safety and Risks of Acetaminophen ...................................... 29
### Overdose Symptoms .............................................................. 33
### Overdose Treatment .............................................................. 35
### Long-Term Use and Side Effects ............................................ 36
### Special Considerations for Certain Populations .................. 39
### Use in Children and Adolescents .......................................... 40
### Use in Older Adults ................................................................ 44
### Key Considerations for Older Adults .................................... 45
### Acetaminophen and Drug Interactions ................................ 47
### The Public Health Use of Acetaminophen ............................ 53
### Ongoing Research .................................................................. 58
### Addressing Safety Concerns .................................................. 64
### Conclusion .............................................................................. 66

## THE END .................................................................................. 72

# CHAPTER ONE

# Introduction

Acetaminophen, also known as paracetamol, is one of the most widely used medicines in the world, introduced as an analgesic and antipyretic agent in the clinical scenario. Few know the history, mechanisms, benefits, and risks of acetaminophen. The book provides an in-depth exploration of acetaminophen from its very discovery up to the current role it plays in modern medicine.

## Early Origins

History has it that the creation of acetaminophen dates back to the 19th century in the quest to find treatments for lowering temperature and relief of pain. The discovery of acetaminophen is accredited by trials of creating alternatives to other analgesics, such as aspirin, which despite its effectiveness, showed many adverse reactions on the user, like stomach irritation and bleeding.

In the late 1800s, chemists have been looking at the derivative of aniline—a collection of group of organic compounds for potential medical use. A good example would be acetanilide, which proved to be an antipyretic, however had a toxic effect on the blood. These studies led to the discovery of phenacetin as yet another derivative with lesser toxicity but still with two important activities—analgesic and antipyretic action.

# The Birth of Acetaminophen

Acetaminophen was first synthesized in 1893 by the French chemist Charles Frédéric Gerhardt, but the medical community did not generally embrace it until the 1940s as a relatively safe and over-the-counter substitute for phenacetin. Scientists had found that acetaminophen was an active metabolite of both acetanilide and phenacetin; thus, it was seen that the body simply converted these compounds into acctaminophen.

Phenacetin was eventually withdrawn because of its

association with kidney damage and other toxic effects, and acetaminophen was widely adopted as a safer alternative. In the 1950s, acetaminophen finally entered the commercial market in the United States, where it quickly achieved tremendous popularity.

# Global Adoption

Over the years, acetaminophen spread wide across the globe in the 20th century. It has been a drug of choice in the management of mild to moderate pain and raising the body temperature, with particular interest shown in its use among children and in a population that portrays gastrointestinal sensitivity with NSAIDs like aspirin.

The creep of acetaminophen into dominance was also supported by the accessible development of OTC formulations that made it available to all without a prescription. Tylenol in

America and Panadol in the United Kingdom are very famous brands that have effectively established the seat of acetaminophen in the world of analgesics.

## Mechanism of Action

Despite its widespread use for many years, the exact

mechanism of action of acetaminophen has been somewhat elusive. It is known that acetaminophen works in the central nervous system, rather than at the site of pain, as do many other analgesics.

Acetaminophen is believed to work by inhibiting, particularly COX-2, an enzyme within the brain. This is said to lead to a reduction in the synthesis of prostaglandins, chemicals that provoke inflammation, pain, and fever. However, acetaminophen does not significantly affect COX-1 such as in NSAIDs, which are rather the cause of its lacking anti-inflammatory actions and its having no irritation effects on the gastrointestinal system.

Recent studies have also determined the probable action of acetaminophen in the modulation of the endocannabinoid system and activation of serotonin pathways in the brain, accounting for its analgesic and antipyretic effects.

## Metabolism and Excretion

Acetaminophen is rapidly and well absorbed from the gastrointestinal tract following oral ingestion. The main site of metabolism is the liver. Conjugation with sulfate and glucuronide converts it to inactive metabolites. A minute portion of acetaminophen is metabolized by the cytochrome P450 enzyme system, more specifically CYP2E1, to a highly reactive molecule called N-Acetyl para benzo-quinone imine, abbreviated as NAPQI.

NAPQI is potentially toxic, although under normal conditions, it gets quickly detoxified by glutathione, a naturally occurring antioxidant of liver origin. The now inactive metabolites, together with the minute amount of unchanged acetaminophen, are then cleared in the urine.

# Pharmacokinetics

The lifetimes of acetaminophen in the body are relatively short, generally between 1 and 4 h in the healthy adult. This means that it is removed fairly rapidly from the body, explaining why the dose can be repeated every 4-6 h to maintain its action on pain or fever.

The onset of action is within 30-60 minutes after ingestion, peak plasma concentrations are reached within 1-2 hours. Duration of action, in general, lasts up to 4-6 hours, making it suitable for acute symptoms.

# Therapeutic Uses of Acetaminophen

Acetaminophen is widely used in the treatment of mild to moderate pain. Its versatility makes this the optimum drug to be used for various conditions like:

Acetaminophen can help relieve tension headaches and migraines. It is good for aching muscles, joints, and the back. This is particularly useful in those patients who cannot tolerate the gastrointestinal problems of NSAIDs.

The usual prescribing dentist may give acetaminophen to

relieve mild to moderate pain following a dental extraction or root canal.

Many women will use acetaminophen to help alleviate the pain of dysmenorrhea, or menstrual cramps.

Only antipyretic considered one of the most widely used.

Taking acetaminophen for

fever is the most probable thing not to induce any gastrointestinal side effect compared to other NSAIDs like aspirin and ibuprofen.

Taking acetaminophen is still the preferred type of fever management, especially in children and even in little children below six months of age. This is because it is safe if properly administered.

## Co-administration with Other Medications

It is done to potentiates its activity or to manage a multitude of symptoms. Some common drug combinations include

Caffeine is combined with acetaminophen to potentiate its analgesic effects. Specifically, it is used for headaches and migraines. Acetaminophen is often combined with an opioid, like codeine or hydrocodone, for the relief of more severe pain, such as postoperative pain or pain caused by cancer.

Acetaminophen is an active ingredient in many multi-symptom cold and flu products; it is combined with a decongestant, antihistamine, and cough suppressant.

# CHAPTER TWO

## Safety and Risks of Acetaminophen

Though relatively safe when used correctly, it is important to stick to the right dosages of acetaminophen to avoid potential risks. Acetaminophen has a maximum recommended daily dose for an adult; it is usually 4,000 milligrams (mg), but according to some professionals, an intake of 3,000 mg is further advised in order to reduce the possibility of liver damage.

With children, one will usually be calculating doses based on weight, possibly in conjunction with age. A caregiver should use a pediatric formulation and should follow the dosing information on the label or as prescribed by a healthcare provider.

One of the major risks related to acetaminophen is overdose, which may cause severe damage to the liver and even death. According to medical statistics, overdose with this very compound is one of the largest causes of acute liver failure in several countries, taking place quite unintentionally.

# Overdose Symptoms

Acetaminophen related overdose symptoms are not felt in the first few hours. Still, thereafter, these include:

Nausea and Vomiting; these are the most common and often the first signs of overdose. Pain in the upper right quadrant of the abdomen may indicate injury to the liver. As the liver begins to fail, concentrations of toxins increase in the blood, leading to confusion, drowsiness, and coma.

A yellow discoloration of the skin and eyes may be a sign of severe liver failure.

## Overdose Treatment

If the patient overdoses on acetaminophen, run them to the hospital immediately. In cases of overdose with acetaminophen, the antidote is N-acetylcysteine, which replenishes the levels of glutathione in the liver to start the detoxification of NAPQI. N-acetylcysteine is most effective when given within 8 to 10 hours after overdose.

## Long-Term Use and Side Effects

Long-term use of acetaminophen, especially in high doses, will also cause hepatic damage. Combining chronic alcohol use with the use of acetaminophen magnifies the risk of liver toxicity because alcohol is an inducer of the CYP2E1 enzyme, leading to an increase in the production of the toxic metabolite NAPQI.

Some studies have suggested that long-term, high-dose acetaminophen therapy may also be associated with other health hazards in addition to hepatic toxicity, including renal damage and gastrointestinal toxicity. These adverse events, however, are generally less than with NSAIDs.

# Special Considerations for Certain Populations

Acetaminophen is one of the safest pain relievers and fever reducers during pregnancy and while breastfeeding. It should, however, be used carefully and under the guidance of a doctor.

# Use in Children and Adolescents

One of the most frequently used drugs in pediatric care is acetaminophen, mainly due to its safe profile and efficiency in the treatment of pain and fever in children.

Most pediatric dosing is based on weight and/or age. Parents or caregivers can use the dosing that appears on the product label or as recommended by a health-care professional to dose the child. Pediatric dosage forms, such as suspensions and chewable tablets, enhance the possibility of easy administration to young children.

The appropriate measuring device included with the medication should be used when giving medication. Parents should be cautioned not to give more than one medication with acetaminophen at the same time to avoid accidental acetaminophen overdose.

Adolescents can usually take adult dosages of acetaminophen. As with the earlier age group, the dosage should be based on body weight. Adolescents, like younger children, should be warned about the dangers of an acetaminophen overdose, particularly if they take the medication on their own.

## Use in Older Adults

Elderly patients are more vulnerable to the possible adverse effects of drugs, including acetaminophen. On the other hand, however, acetaminophen is usually preferred to NSAIDs because of the lesser potential for gastrointestinal bleeding and kidney damage.

## Key Considerations for Older Adults

Although the adult dose is generally considered safe for

elderly patients, clinicians may prescribe a lower dosage, particularly for those patients with hepatic or renal failure. The elderly also ought to be observed for liver toxicity, especially during concomitant administration with drugs that inhibit liver functions and among habitual alcohol users.

# Acetaminophen and Drug Interactions

Acetaminophen is very well tolerated and has very few drug-to-drug interactions relative to the other analgesic medications. Nevertheless, a few interactions may be found.

Chronic alcohol use increases the risk of liver injury when combined with acetaminophen. Chronic use of ethanol induces the enzyme CYP2E1, creating an increase in the production of the toxic metabolite NAPQI. Heavy drinkers are cautioned to avoid therapeutic doses of acetaminophen and advised to consult a healthcare professional before consumption.

Warfarin is an anticoagulant that works to keep you from building up blood clots. Acetaminophen can potentiate the anticoagulant effect of warfarin and enhance the risk of bleeding. People taking warfarin should exercise caution in using acetaminophen and be closely monitored by an INR at regular intervals.

Drugs that induce an increase in the activity of liver enzymes—for example, phenytoin, carbamazepine, and rifampin—lead to an increased acetaminophen metabolism toward the toxic metabolite NAPQI. Patients on such treatments are particularly at more increased risk once they experience toxicity.

Cholestyramine, a bile acid sequestrant used to lower cholesterol, decreases the absorption of acetaminophen, thus lowering the effect.

Acetaminophen should be given 1 hour before or 4 hours after cholestyramine administration.

Other herbal supplements, such as St. John's Wort, are strong liver enzyme inducers and will cause different metabolism of the acetaminophen. Patients on herbal supplements require informing the health care provider to assess for interactions.

## The Public Health Use of Acetaminophen

The public health importance attached to acetaminophen is great, serving as the only treatment available to the general public for fever, relieving pain, and being a very effective treatment. Acetaminophen has been widely used as an over-the-counter medication to be a very valuable asset in self-care and pain management.

Acetaminophen is an over-the-counter drug, and this status has caused it to become one of the most used drugs in the world. It comes in different forms such as tablets, capsules, liquid suspensions, and suppositories, hence it is accessible to humans across all age groups- young to old, and even to the handicapped.

It is a reasonably inexpensive drug, hence reasonably affordable even to low- and middle-income countries, for both pain relief and temperature.

Public Health Campaigns

Public health campaigns have been carried out to make

people aware of the safe use of acetaminophen, especially adhering to recommended dosages and looking for overdose symptoms.

Attempts have been made regarding safe medication practice, likc proper storage and labeling of medications, to avoid accidental overdose in children.

# Ongoing Research

Years of application have passed and still, the research and development of acetaminophen are underway. As of now, the work of scientists on this medication has managed to divert in another direction: the mechanisms of action, new therapeutic uses, and ways in which risks associated with it can be reduced.

However, research is still ongoing to definitively establish the exact pathways through which acetaminophen works as an analgesic and an antipyretic. Breakthroughs in molecular biology and pharmacology may open new dimensions about the interaction of acetaminophen with the different pathways in the body, maybe resulting in the development and innovation of new targeted options for pain management. Of major interest is the interaction between acetaminophen and the endocannabinoid system, which is responsible for pain modulation. Deciphering such interactions could offer new avenues for the development of therapy in pain management that takes advantage of acetaminophen benefits, with fewer associated risks.

Another line on which development is focused is extended-release drug formulations of acetaminophen that offer prolonged pain relief while reducing dosing frequency. It is aimed at enhancing patient compliance while minimizing the risk of overdose.

Such innovative combination therapies that have paracetamol combined with other analgesics or adjuvants are under investigation, as they might provide strong pain relief while reducing side effects. Such combinations might especially become very valuable in the treatment of chronic pain conditions.

# Addressing Safety Concerns

Recently, there have been efforts to develop strategies for decreasing the potential risk of liver toxicity associated with acetaminophen, including the identification of biomarkers for the susceptibility of a given individual to toxicity and the development of adjunct therapies that might reduce the potential toxic effect of the drug on the liver. These also include public health interventions in order to reduce the incidence of acetaminophen overdose. These include improvement in packaging and labeling, public awareness, and the formulation of guidelines for health practitioners to ensure safe prescription principles.

## Conclusion

Acetaminophen was initially discovered over 100 years ago and is now a common trusted method of pain and fever management in millions of people around the world. Yet, acetaminophen is not without its risks and an appreciation of its pharmacology, therapeutic uses, safety, and future directions for current and future patients and overall health care providers is imperative.

As good as this drug is, there is more knowledge coming on this drug, and further public health initiatives and research will continue to help this great drug, acetaminophen, to be both safe and effective in our medical arsenal.

By balancing benefits with caution and prudent use, we can continue to rely upon this invaluable medication for generations to come.

# THE END

www.ingramcontent.com/pod-product-compliance
Lightning Source LLC
Chambersburg PA
CBHW070212230526
45471CB00002B/935